# YOGA
## within

# YOGA
## within

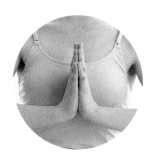

By CARRIE SCHNEIDER

Photographs by ERICKA McCONNELL

Stewart, Tabori & Chang
New York

Published in 2001 by
Stewart, Tabori & Chang
A Company of La Martinière Groupe
115 West 18th Street
New York, NY 10011

Library of Congress Cataloging-in-Publication Data

Schneider, Carrie
Yoga within / by Carrie Schneider; photography by Ericka McConnell.
p. cm.
ISBN 1-58479-123-3
1. Yoga, Hatha. 2. Yoga—Philosophy. I. Title.

RA781.7.S298 2001
613.7'046—dc21
2001032826

The text of this book was composed in Trebuchet.
Printed in Singapore

10 9 8 7 6 5 4 3 2 1

First Printing

## Contributors

DESIGN AND ART DIRECTION: Nina Barnett
EDITORS: Sandra Gilbert and Emily Von Kohorn
PRODUCTION MANAGER: Kim Tyner

PHOTOGRAPHER: Ericka McConnell
PHOTOGRAPHY ASSISTANTS: Nettie Rencher, Buff Strickland

MODELS (page 6, from left to right): Paul Hudson, Kristin McGee, Heath House, Cynthia Bueschel

MAKEUP AND HAIR: Elisa A. Flowers

STYLIST: Samantha Strauss
WARDROBE AND ACCESSORIES: courtesy of Crunch, Jacques Moret, Jivamukti Yoga Center

## Bibliography

p. 7 Dylan Thomas, "The Force That Through the Green Fuse Drives the Flower," *The Norton Anthology of Modern Poetry*, ed. Richard Ellmann and Robert O'Clair (New York and London: W. W. Norton and Company, 1988), 920. Copyright © by New Directions, N.Y.
p. 20 Lao Tsu, *The Tao Te Ching*, trans. Gia-fu Feng and Jane English (New York: Vintage Books Edition, 1977), 18.
p. 31 B.K.S. Iyengar, *Light on Yoga* (New York: Schocken Books, 1979), 35-36 (abridged quote).
p. 32 *The I Ching or Book of Changes*, trans. Richard Wilhelm (Princeton, N.J.: Princeton University Press, 1977), 133-34.
p. 37 *The Bhagavad Gita*, trans. Stephen Mitchell (New York: Harmony Books, a division of Random House, Inc., 2000), 92. Copyright © 2000 by Stephen Mitchell.
p. 43 T.K.V. Desikachar, *The Heart of Yoga: Developing a Personal Practice* (Rochester, Vt.: Inner Traditions International, 1995), 159.
p. 47 Swami Vivekananda, *Meditation and Its Methods* (Calcutta: Advaita Ashram Publication Department, 1991), 83.
p. 54 Swami Sivananda, *Epistles of Swami Sivananda* (Shivanandanagar: Divine Life Society, 1968), 37.
p. 57 J. Krishnamurti, *On Love and Loneliness* (New York: HarperCollins Publishers, 1993), 2.
p. 74 Vivekananda, 83.
p. 76 Paramahansa Yogananda, *Autobiography of a Yogi* (Los Angeles: Self-Realization Fellowship, 1974), 280.
p. 77 Sivananda, 23.
p. 79 Pema Chödrön, *The Wisdom of No Escape and the Path of Loving-Kindness*. (Boston: Shambala Publications, 1991), 46-47.

Every effort has been made to trace copyright holders of material in this book.

*To my teachers,
beginning with Marty and Ruth*

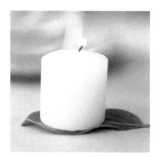

I am indebted to the people who helped make this book possible. At Stewart, Tabori & Chang, thanks to Leslie Stoker, for keeping me on her Rolodex; to Sandra Gilbert, for entertaining and making good on the notion; to Nina Barnett, for her interested eye; and to Emily Von Kohorn, for patience and fortitude. Endless appreciation for the support editorial and otherwise of Jon Cassota, Hilary Fulton, Michael Hutchison, Lisa Landphair, Jim Paisner, and Christopher Widney. Gratitude to Nancy Vinik for lighting the match, to Stephen Cope for fanning the fire, and to Peter Thomashow and Henry Sapoznik for tending it awhile. And big-time pranams to Cynthia Bueschel, Heath House, Paul Hudson, and Kristin McGee, whose beauty and love of yoga grace these pages.

The light within me salutes the light within you.

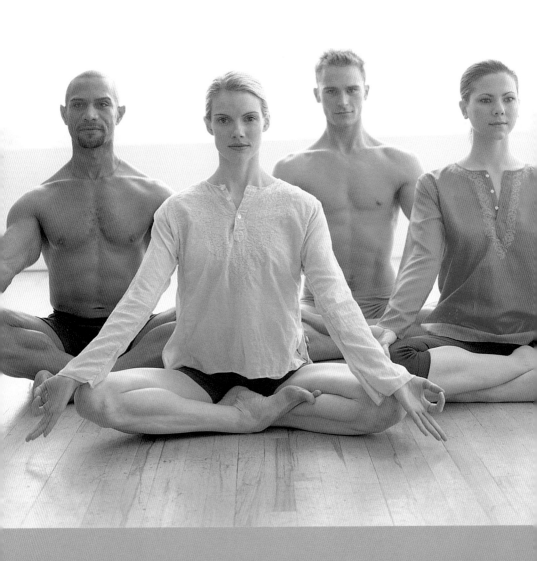

# Approaching Yoga Within

What "yoga" means has been as variously proclaimed as the names for God. From the Sanskrit *yuj*, or yoke, the word itself translates as "to join" or "to be joined with," and from there the interpretations somersault over one another until they rejoin themselves. The ability to direct the mind without distraction, the state of wholeness, the control of thought-waves, union with the divine—all these definitions describe the goal of the ancient physical, philosophical, mental, and spiritual disciplines collectively known as yoga.

As we move through the shapes of yoga *asanas*—the postures that comprise its physical practice—we are perceptibly moved and shaped by them. Exercises like the ones in this book systematically stretch then contract, strengthen then relax targeted muscle groups and internal organs, bringing us to new levels of health, fitness, and mental acuity.

But *hatha* (forceful) yoga postures are a means to a distinctly nonphysical end: to realize our connection with "the force that through the green fuse drives the flower," as the eminent yogi Dylan Thomas so finely phrased it. The Welsh poet would likely be surprised by this honorific; he was not an Indian philosopher and almost certainly never draped his ankle over his head. But in writing lines like the one above, Thomas practiced yoga. When Miles Davis blew heartbreakingly beautiful riffs on his horn, he "did" yoga. When you are able to quiet the chatter in the mind—moving past "I want," "I need," "I have," "I don't have," "I wish I didn't have," "what if I don't get"—and for seconds or minutes at a time can exist in this moment now instead of being subsumed by memory or expectation, you approach yoga within.

The practice of yoga lifts the cloud of *avidya*—misperception—so that we may see and act and live more correctly. The *asanas*, when we first begin them, hint at what we have forgotten. They are whispers down the corridor we are glad to hear again. So we learn to listen closely, through more *asana* and or through another of the eight avenues to the state of yoga explored in these pages.

Perhaps you found your way to *asana* practice to get thinner thighs and a nice butt—which you will, if you stick with it. But if you stick with it, the other seven routes to yoga will almost certainly find their way to you. Yoga philosophy's personal and social observances, the *yamas* and *niyamas*, heighten our function in the world around us. *Asana* affords us greater comfort within the embodied state. *Pranayama*, breath expansion, harnesses and lets us be harnessed by the life force within us. *Pratyahara*, sense withdrawal, frees us from servitude to the vagaries of what we perceive. These five disciplines together hone our minds to *dharana*, the ability to concentrate—on *asana*, on mantra, on any one thing, on one everything. Concentration enables meditation, *dhyana*, the chance to spend time with the supreme intelligence we otherwise just dance with on occasion. And all seven routes lead to *samadhi*, absorption with that intelligence.

Ancient Sanskrit texts from the *Vedas* to the *Yoga Sutras* chart the way to the destination based on adherence to principles that generally lie at the core of all world religions. Yoga is not a religion, however, so whether you invoke divine energy as Yaweh, Allah, Buddha, God, Isvara, Om, or none of the above, you can embrace and be embraced by its practice.

*Yoga Within* juxtaposes these principles and observances with poses that lend themselves to their examination. Selected images and text excerpts will allow you to use this tool again and again as you deepen your journey to the state of yoga.

"*Yogasgcittavrttinirodhah*," the second aphorism in the *Yoga Sutras*, tells us that yoga stills the vicissitudes of the mind. This is not to say you should negate joy and sorrow, eagerness and reluctance, but rather that you can become awakened to how emotions color perceptions. By watching our reactions shape our actions, we begin to grasp *kaivalya*, or freedom, with open hands, the only way it will be held.

# SADHANA

That which we can practice

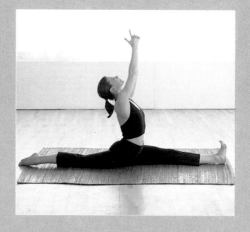

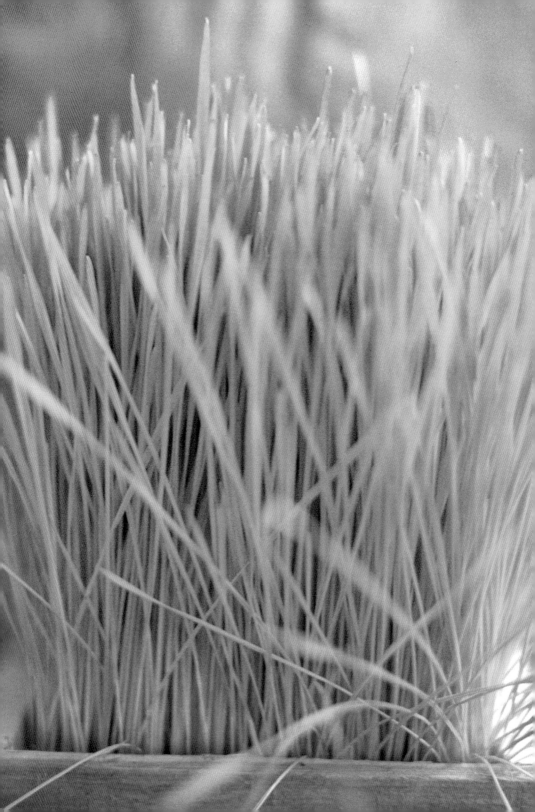

# Sun Salutation (Surya Namaskar)

When we salute the sun, a common beginning of *asana* practice, we warm to the radiance of healthful mobility by stretching ourselves in every direction. But the thread here, as for all postures flowing and held, is the breath. Before you begin moving your body, observe the movement of your breath. Take time to wonder at this involuntary reflex that so reflects volition. Breath happens inside you, but it does not originate there. You do not create it. Where does it come from?

As you step, lift, and press through the following postures, continue to watch the breath, which in yoga practice is as much bellwether as bodily function. By using the method of *ujjayi* (victory) breathing, accomplished by slightly constricting the throat passage, each inhalation and exhalation through the nose is an audible whisper, like the steady, unending sound of the ocean. Follow these whispers until they become a metronome and a gauge of the flow of *prana*, life force energy, within. And if you feel the pace quicken or stop, or if what you hear is less a whisper than a growl or a groan, back off a tad until you regain the steady, deep, even rhythm you experience in repose or concentration.

We move sequentially through the shapes of *Surya Namaskar*—like all *asanas*, patterned on and named for animals, natural phenomena, or the supernatural qualities they invoke—with as little as one breath per movement. Continued throughout an entire *asana* session, this style of practice has been dubbed *vinyasa* yoga, the sweaty, nearly aerobic approach that increasingly defines the American brand of the discipline.

Fashioned on the muscular ballet of *astanga*, a fast-moving series of postures strung together with gymnastic-style jumps and balances, *vinyasa* yoga classes challenge the body and mind while teaching grace and agility. But much remains to be learned from the slower, more circumspect *hatha* yoga practices first brought to these shores in the early 1900s. Our charge, then, is to imbue the most action-packed health club "power" yoga class with the unhurried intelligence of what was practiced in Himalayan caves five thousand years ago. As twenty-first-century Americans, our influences are myriad. We are generally not Hindu, nor need we be to incorporate the tenets of yoga philosophy. Take what you choose and leave the rest to find you, as it does. And let *Surya Namaskar*, like your entire yoga practice, lead you where you become ready to go.

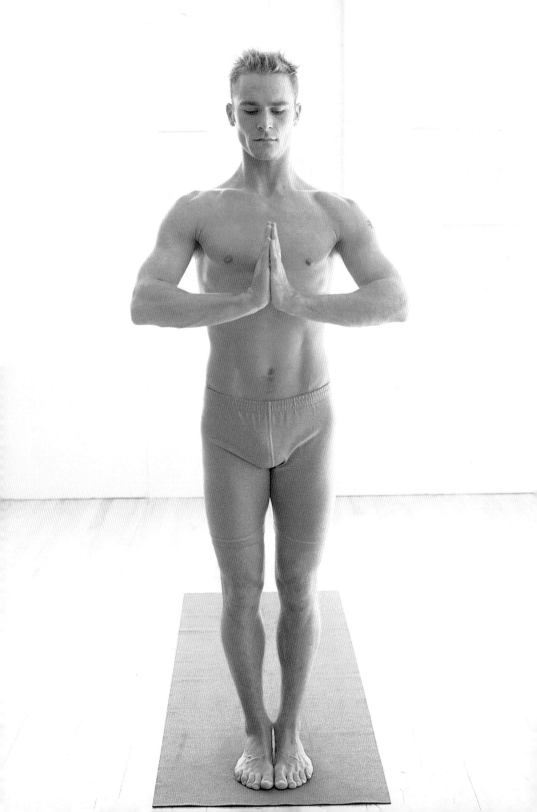

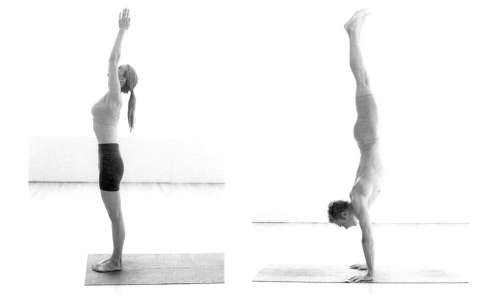

## Mountain (Tadasana)

Coming to stand in *Tadasana*, we align ourselves anew at the start of each practice. Press the insides of your feet together and grow sensate through the soles, spreading the weight and skin evenly onto the floor. As you move awareness up the legs, hug bone with muscle until you come to tighten the pelvic floor, then settle into the lifting energy that provides. Raise arms overhead with palms together in prayer, pulling navel toward spine and sending the tailbone to the floor as the crown of the head reaches to the ceiling. Stand to your full measure with the solemn power and quiet strength of a mountain, the inspiration for this posture.

Whether you are standing up, upside down, sideways, or on one leg, the centered alignment of *Tadasana* lies at the core of all *asanas*. Find it in every pose. Above, Handstand (*Adho Mukha Vrksasana*).

**DRISHTI (GAZE):** The eyes, portals of the soul, can dart about, anxious to take in all they can. They can settle languorously, engendering sloth. In yoga practice, keep the gaze softly attentive—fixed directly before you, at the tip of your nose, or upward, depending on the posture, but always open, alert, relaxed, ready. Look at nothing in particular; see everything supremely.

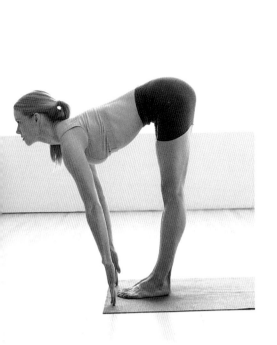 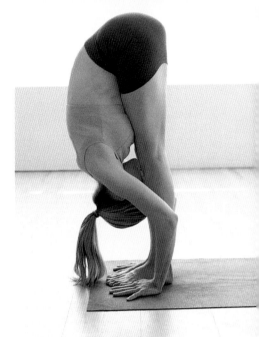

# Extreme Forward Bend (Uttanasana)

With the chest open, not caved in, swan dive to the floor, then rise to finger-tips or higher to flatten the back and straighten the legs. Keep weight toward the balls of the feet with the front legs actively engaged so you do not rock back in the heels, which hyperextends the knee joints and stresses the hamstrings. Look forward, lengthening head away from sitting bones, and retain that length as you fold deep into the posture, fingers in line with toes, palms to floor if possible. (Learn what this feels like, even if you need to bend your knees.)

In addition to stretching the legs, forward bends are about elongating the spine. Let your head and neck hang heavy, as if lead weights are attached at the shoulders, until the drape of your torso straightens your legs. Lift where the hamstrings and sitting bones meet, and as you exhale pull navel toward spine, making room to bend deeply.

Next, move into a lunge by stepping your right foot back as far as it will go with the left knee bent ninety degrees over the ankle. Rise to fingertips and stretch the back of the right knee open by activating the quadriceps and pressing strongly and evenly into the whole foot, buttressing stretch with strength. Radiate one line of energy from the heel to the crown of the head.

Avoid joint injury by securing right-angle alignment in all single bent-knee standing postures.

A house cannot stand without a firm, solidly constructed foundation. Build your *asanas* with care. Employ correct alignment from the get-go, so you can discern the larger meaning of their practice.

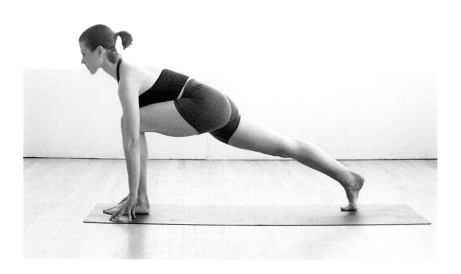

# Four-Limbed Staff (Chaturanga Dandasana)

Press your left foot back to meet your right until your body is one solid plank of energy. Check to see that your palms are directly under your shoulders and your feet are as far behind you as they can go, so the buttocks neither sag nor poke up. Keep sending energy through the heels as you bend your elbows directly back—not out—and lower the plank until you hover above the floor.

This pose can be daunting for new practitioners, especially for women who initially lack the upper-body strength more inherent in the male physique. A good preparation is to drop the knees, chest, and chin to the floor, keeping the hips raised, like an inchworm. But also try moving from plank into the *Chaturanga* you are able to do now, bending your elbows back one inch today, lowering to eight inches off the floor tomorrow—or next year.

**VAIRAGYA (FREEDOM FROM WANTING):** There is always someplace to go in yoga; the trick is to be where you are now. Diligence produces surprisingly rapid results. Still, learn to observe progress in postures with dispassion, not lingering in satisfaction once you reach a goal. If you can raise your foot to your ear, you'll soon meet someone who tucks both feet handily around his head. The lesson is that accomplishment can bring as much unhappiness as failure. Become attached to neither. Let work be its own reward.

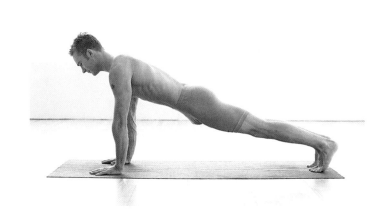

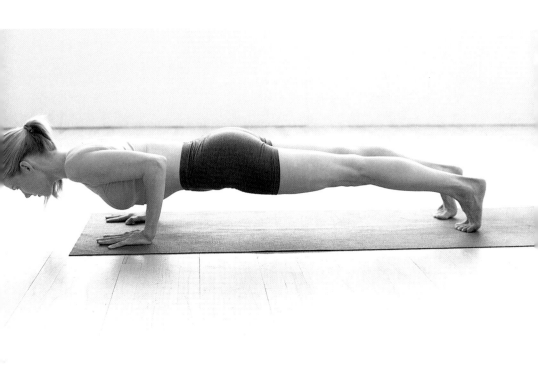

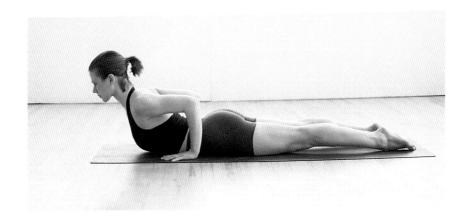

## Cobra (Bhujangasana)

With palms alongside the chest, elbows over wrists, slowly raise head, neck, and chest off the floor in such a way that the lower ribs stay down and you can lift your hands. Keep the neck in line with the spine and press the tops of the feet into the floor so strongly the kneecaps lift. Spread your pinky toes and feel how this translates into a broadening across the sacrum, your protection against lower-back pain.

## Upward-Facing Dog (Urdhva Mukha Svanasana)

On an inhale, press the arms straight and pull the chest forward and up until the hips and thighs lift, coming to balance on the palms and tops of the feet. Stretch your legs away behind you.

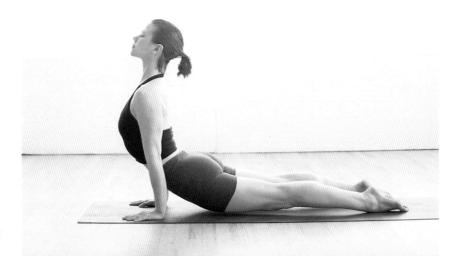

# Downward-Facing Dog (Adho Mukha Svanasana)

Raise your hips to the ceiling on an exhale by pushing into the heels of the hands and feet, forming an upside-down V. People who've been practicing for twenty-five years say Downdog never stops changing for them; see how it evolves for you as you refine the posture internally and externally. Rotate the upper inner thighs in and back. Send the heels down and press into all ten fingers, especially the thumbs and first knuckle of the forefingers. Establish a straight line of energy from hips to shoulders, bending knees if necessary to feel that. Roll upper arms and inner elbows out, shoulder blades down the back. Look toward your navel; if the ribcage hangs down, draw it in by taking more weight back in the hips and using the arms and legs more strongly.

Stay in the pose at least five breaths, then complete *Surya Namaskar*: Step right then left foot to the hands; inhale, lift the heart, look up; exhale, fold into the legs; inhale, circle the arms out and up as you dive to the ceiling and press the palms overhead; exhale the arms alongside the body to *Tadasana*. Repeat on the left side, moving through three to five complete cycles per side. (You may also choose to jump back to *Chaturanga* and forward to *Uttanasana*, intensifying the *vinyasa* aspect of Sun Salutations.)

Animals stretch themselves this way all the time; learn what they know intrinsically about maintaining the health and purpose of muscle, joint, and ligament to awaken and celebrate life-force energy.

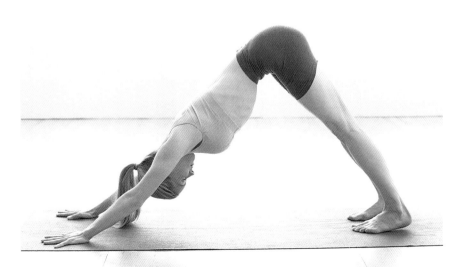

The newborn's infectious beauty is her untarnished reflection of *Atman*, divinity within. Regain the sense of wonder in which she is immersed. Move through these postures as a joyous witness, free from the shackles of expectation and anticipation.

*Carrying body and soul and embracing the one,*
*Can you avoid separation?*
*Attending fully and becoming supple,*
*Can you be as a newborn babe?*
*Understanding and being open to all things,*
*Are you able to do nothing?*
*Giving birth and nourishing,*
*Bearing yet not possessing,*
*Working yet not taking credit,*
*Leading yet not dominating,*
*This is the Primal Virtue.*

—Lao Tsu, *Tao Te Ching*

**S A T Y A  ( T R U T H )**: "Beauty is truth, truth beauty," wrote John Keats, another yogi of a poet. That line of poetry is writ large and new in the face of every child. It is as evident in yoga philosophy, which advocates *satya* in thought, communication, action, and deed.

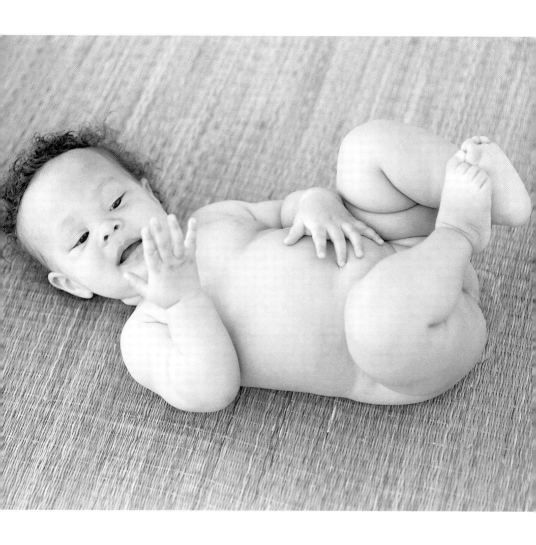

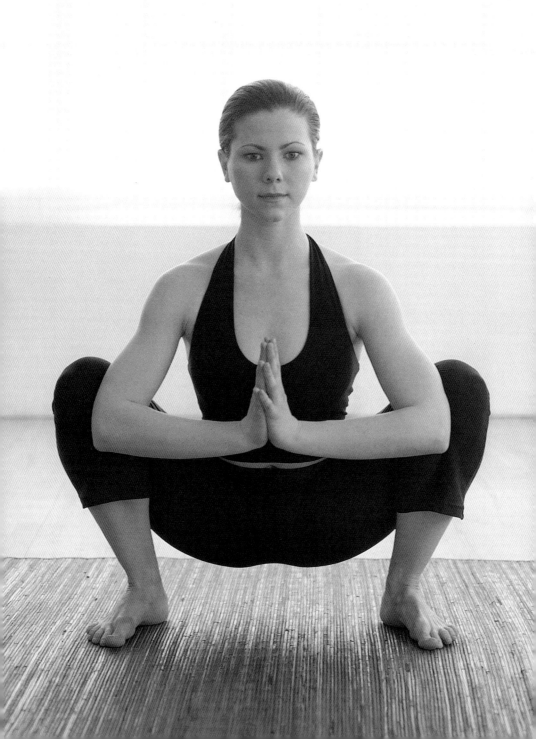

In non-Western cultures people often sit on their haunches, an organic seating arrangement Westerners eschew, reducing the hip and knee joints' natural function. Reclaim this fundamental ability through the variety of *asanas* built on and around it.

**TAPAS (IGNITION):** Performing *asanas* and spiritual disciplines intensively fuels purification of body and mind. *Utkatasana* moves us out of the concept and into the fire. Keep cool.

## Fierce Seat (Utkatasana)

Pressing feet, knees, and thighs together and heels down, sit deeply while raising the torso and arms up as much as possible. Tighten the perineum— the muscle between the anus and genitals—to keep your seat without swaying the back or jutting the ribs forward. Relax your shoulders down the back, reducing tension there and everywhere.

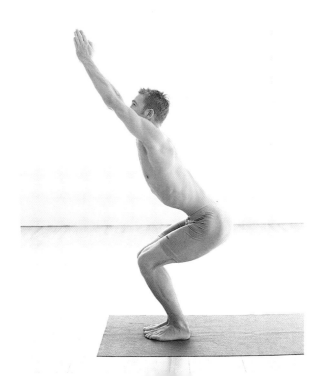

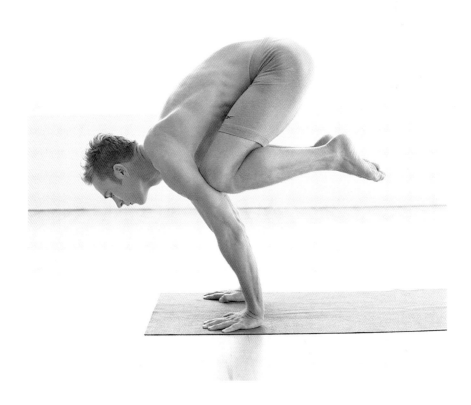

The whole world—and our existence within it—spins on the cycling of three qualities of nature, known in yoga philosophy as the *gunas*: *sattva* (clarity), *rajas* (compulsion toward movement), and *tamas* (resistance toward advancement). The balance of our perceptions is eternally tipped by these forces, but the yogi grows quietly attuned to their play, and to its effects.

Note the *gunas* at work as you rise up into Crane pose (*Bakasana*) by propping your knees on the backs of your upper arms until the seat and legs lift. In learning to practice balancing poses with brave curiosity and disregard for the eruptions of *rajas* and *tamas*, we come to rest in the stasis of *sattva*, clarity, yoga.

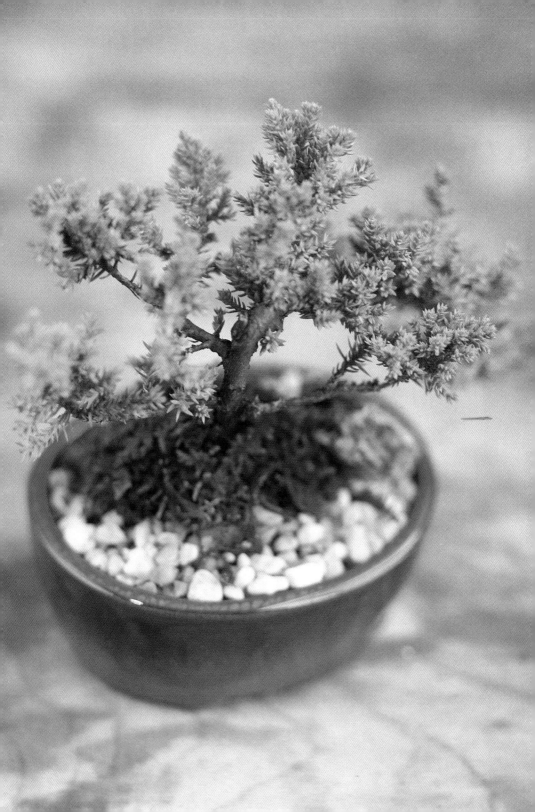

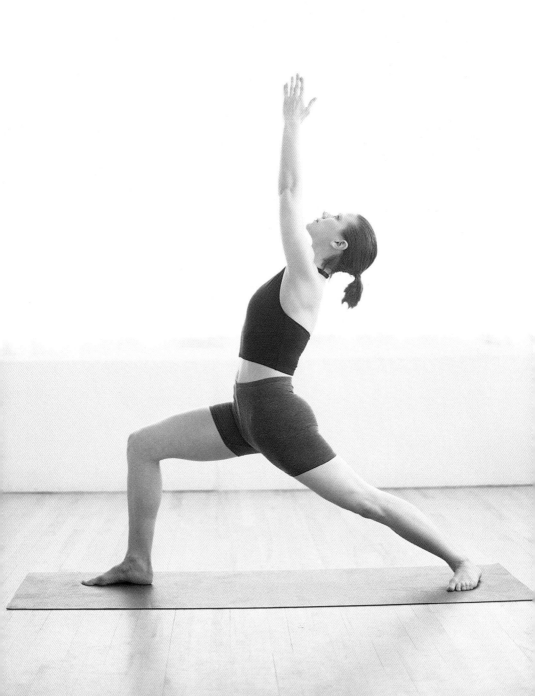

# Warrior One (Virabhadrasana I)

Take "warrior stance": feet one leg length apart with right foot turned out ninety degrees and left foot in forty-five degrees, until right heel aligns with left arch. Bend right knee and turn torso over the thigh, squaring hips forward. Pull your right hip back and press the outer edge of your left foot down to move the left hip forward. Cement this posture's pedestal, holding firm below the navel as you elevate the upper back, arms, and gaze to the ceiling. Work with straight arms, inner elbows reaching toward each other and palms flat together in prayer.

As with all alternate-side postures, hold five to eight breaths and change sides.

Yogis are warriors for peace. If that strikes you as hyperbole, strike this posture deeply and correctly for eight slow breaths and watch the mind. As the front knee bends straight forward and the back foot and leg presses firmly away, your mind may say, "Get me out of here." Stay. Learn what there is to be learned in this and every *asana*.

**SAMSKARAS (IMPRESSIONS):** One intention of yoga practice is to free us from formed patterns of thought and behavior that are no longer—or never were—for the good. How unfortunate it would be if our practice brought about negative *samskaras* of its own! Keep *asana* regularly fresh, instead of rote, by being sweetly attentive in each pose you take. There's nothing new under the sun, the saying goes; but the *Virabhadrasana* you are in now, like this breath you draw, will not happen again. Stay grounded in the moment. Attention to the breath and to details of structure keep us there by keeping us here—an excellent new *samskara* to form.

*sthirasukhamasanam*

—*Yoga Sutras*


*Sthira* is Sanskrit for "steady," *sukha*, "comfortable," and *asana*, "seat." This aphorism, or *sutra*, instructs that postures should be firm but relaxed. By training body and mind to find easy groundedness in each posture, we develop equanimity amid the changing shapes of our lives.

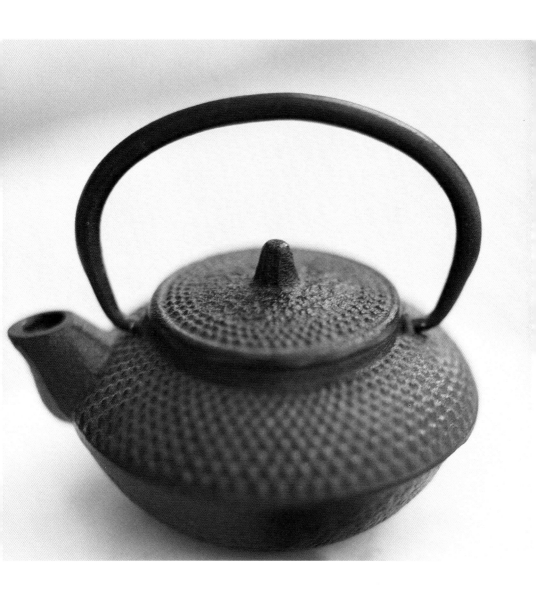

# Warrior Two (Virabhadrasana II)

From warrior stance, press strongly into the outer left leg and foot to bend right knee, this time keeping the chest directly over the hips as they broaden. Extend arms straight out from the shoulders. Gaze out over the back of the right hand and intuit an uninterrupted flow of energy from the left fingertips. Warrior Two is not a backbend; lengthen the tailbone down and toward the pubic bone until your torso rises from the legs and hips like a tree trunk. Feel your great strength, and your great vulnerability.

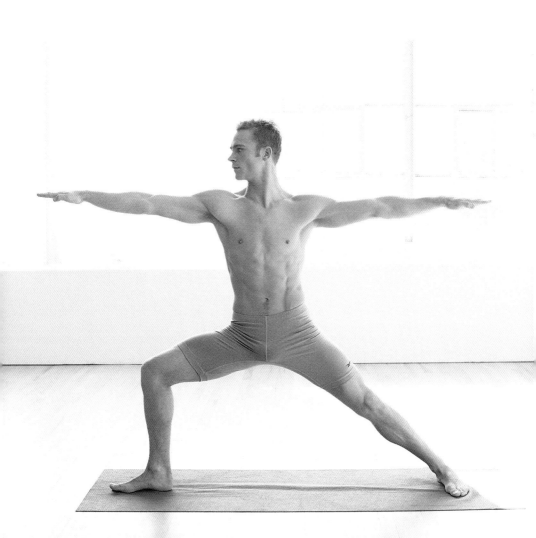

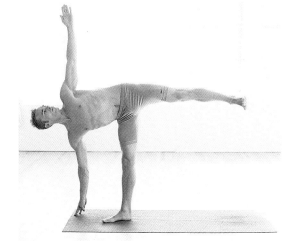

# Half-Moon (Ardha Chandrasana)

With the knee still bent, reach right hand to the floor a foot in front of and to the outside of your right foot, thumb in line with pinky toe. Pressing the right foot and fingertips down, move left foot toward right, straighten right leg and lift left leg directly back out of the hip socket, flexing the foot behind you. Stack left hip on right hip and left shoulder on right shoulder, then see about extending the left arm straight up, gazing at the thumb. Spin your chest to the ceiling.

Slow, deliberate movement is essential to finding balance. Relax into the holding as you observe the dance between musculature and will, alignment and ego.

**NONGRASPING (APARIGRAHA):** *During the dark half of the month, the moon rises late when most men are asleep and so do not appreciate its beauty. Its splendor wanes but it does not stray from its path and is indifferent to man's lack of appreciation. It has faith that it will be full again when it faces the Sun, and then men will eagerly await its glorious rising.*

*The life of an ordinary man is filled with an unending series of disturbances and frustrations and with his reactions to them. Thus there is hardly any possibility of keeping the mind in a state of equilibrium. By the observance of* aparigraha, *another facet of* asteya *(nonstealing), the yogi makes his life as simple as possible and trains his mind not to feel the loss or lack of anything. Then everything he really needs will come to him by itself at the proper time.*

—B.K.S. Iyengar, *Light on Yoga*

Like the Bible, Koran, and Talmud, China's ancient text the *I Ching* (Book of Changes) is a collection of wisdom that frequently parallels yogic literature. The *I Ching*'s teachings are comprised in hexagrams said to describe all possible arrangements of the eternal play of energies. The thirty-fourth hexagram echoes the *Sutras* by cautioning against the sudden desire to act harshly, often the result of lower instincts like anger, possessiveness, and fear.

## TA CHUANG/THE POWER OF THE GREAT

above, *chên*, the arousing, thunder

below, *ch'ien*, the creative, heaven

*The toes are in the lowest place and are ready to advance. So likewise great power in lowly station is inclined to effect advance by force. There is danger that one may rely entirely on one's own power and forget to ask what is right. Too, being intent on movement one may not wait for the right time.*

*Perseverance in equilibrium brings good fortune. Truly great power does not degenerate into mere force but remains inwardly united with the principles of right and of justice. When we understand this point, we understand the true meaning of all that happens in heaven and on earth.*

—*I Ching*

Monitor the wish to leap out of difficult postures. Note the workings of your mind here, which likely resemble your inner dialogue in any tricky situation. Translate the urge to bolt, born of insecurity, into a strength rooted in graceful acceptance. "Perseverance in equilibrium," the *I Ching* and *Sutras* prescribe.

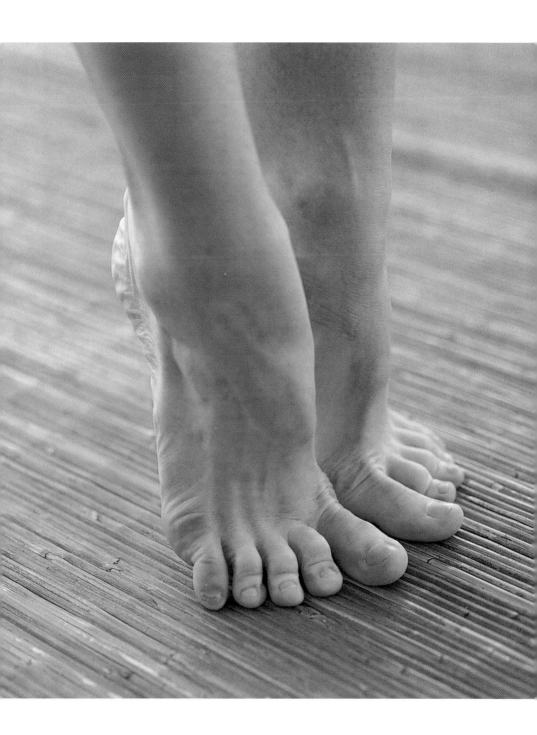

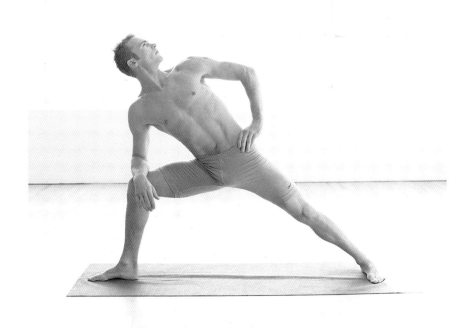

# Extended Side Angle
## (Utthita Parsvakonasana)

From a wide warrior stance, bend the right knee and reach right arm and left and right side of the body to the right. Pressing strongly into the outer left foot and leg, prop right elbow onto right knee and rest forearm on thigh. Reach the left arm over your ear in a long line diagonal with and on the same plane as your left leg. Keep shoulders and chest parallel to the wall in front of you. Where you start to lose that open orientation of the chest and shoulders is where you should stop advancing in the pose.

Look up into your biceps and then into the palm, which faces the floor. Maintaining that gaze as well as the breadth across chest, continue by placing the right fingertips or palm outside your right foot. Roll the right buttock under as you extend from the outer left foot to the left middle finger.

Binding the posture—thread right arm under the thigh and clasp the left wrist behind the back—deepens the twist in the upper back, another instance of freedom emerging from restraint.

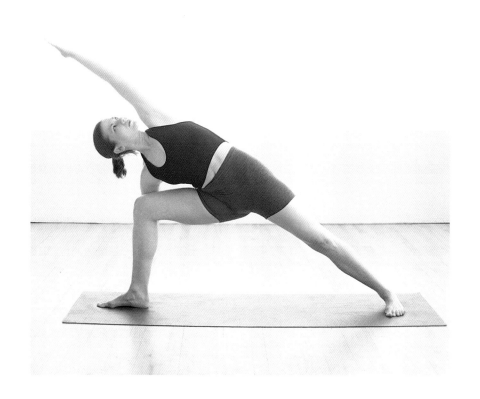

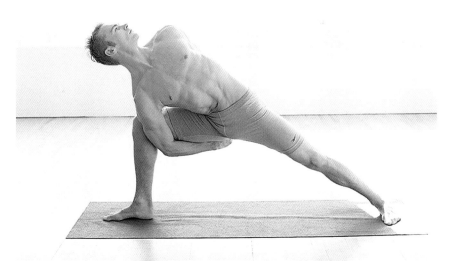

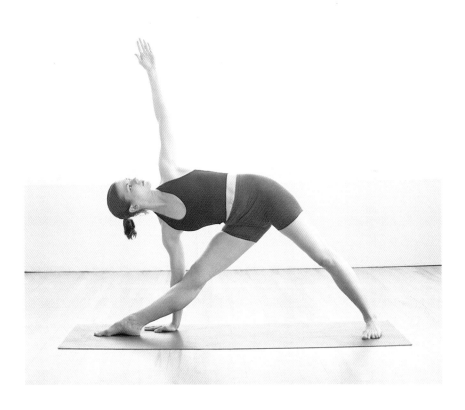

# Triangle (Utthita Trikonasana)

With feet in warrior stance, extend arms straight from the shoulders and
pause a moment, feeling the breadth of your wingspan and strength of your
feet and legs, quadriceps actively contracted. On an inhale, shift the torso as
far to the right as you can and as you exhale, windmill the right arm down
and left arm up. Aim not for the floor but for the heavens: rest your right
hand wherever it lands—on your right ankle or shin or on the floor outside
your foot—and reach the left arm straight out of the shoulder. Don't throw the
arm back further than the eyes can follow; it is the ribs that want to spin,
with the uplifted arm the arbiter rather than initiator of the twist. Lengthen
your head away from the tailbone until the right side of your torso is parallel
to the floor. With each exhalation rotate the left upper back more toward the
wall behind you. Feel energy radiate from right to left hand.

*"A lamp sheltered from the wind
which does not falter"—to this
is compared the true man of yoga
whose mind has vanished in the Self.*

*He knows the infinite joy
that is reached by the understanding
beyond the senses; steadfast,
he does not fall back from the truth.*

*Attaining this state, he knows
that there is no higher attainment.
He is rooted there, unshaken
even by the deepest sorrow.*

*This is true yoga: the unbinding
of the bonds of sorrow. Practice
this yoga with determination
and with a courageous heart.*

*—Bhagavad Gita*

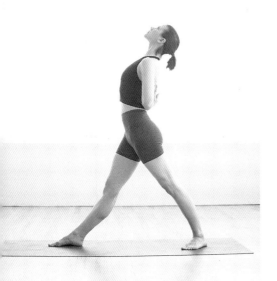
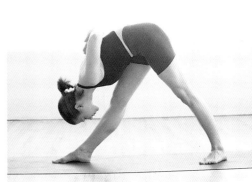

# Extended Flank Stretch (Parsvottanasana)

Step the feet less wide apart than for warrior stance, then angle the left foot in more acutely until the hips and torso square easily over the right leg. With hands on hips, push your middle fingers into the hollows where the torso meets the inner thigh. Feel what goes on as you begin to draw the hips back and send the chest forward. Then raise the torso and fold forward again with palms pressed together behind your back in a prayer, clasping alternate elbows if your palms do not meet. The idea here is to keep the chest open as you bow forward, aiming heart to knee.

**SIDDHIS (POWERS):** By refining sense perception through its deliberate study, the yogi can come to develop *siddhis*, supernatural powers ranging from prescience to the ability to calibrate the metabolism. Students may not walk through the walls at your neighborhood yoga studio, but many practitioners do experience increased occurrences of ESP—"I knew you were going to call!"—as well as a heightened body awareness that advances more than just *asana* practice. Expect nothing; keep an open mind.

# Revolved Triangle (Parivrtta Trikonasana)

From *Parsvottanasana*, lower your left hand to the floor outside your right foot and pull the right hip back, looking up over the shoulder (shown below on opposite side). Initiate a twist from the mid to upper back, then extend the right arm up and feel the same expansion across the chest as you do in Triangle.

Like a pup tent, Revolved Triangle cannot stand unless each point of its tripod base is firmly staked in the earth. Press into the hand, the front big toe ball joint, and the outer edge of the back foot. If your hand does not reach the floor, raise the floor to meet it by using a block or a phonebook. Be patient as you teach yourself this pose, which is both a balance and a twist. Vary your approach: Bend the front knee to get your hand down; use a prop and keep the front leg straight; or stay and grow more comfortable in the previous pose, an excellent preparation for *Parivrtta Trikonasana*.

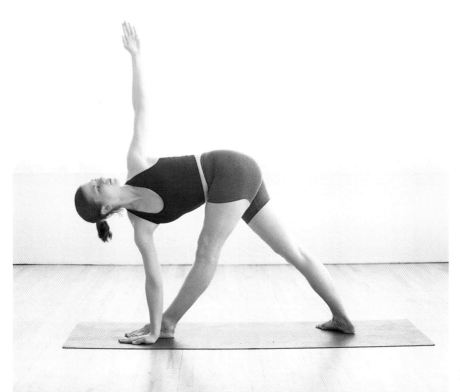

# Peacock Feather (Pincha Mayurasana)

From a kneeling position, hug your elbows on the floor beneath your shoulders and extend the forearms straight forward with palms down and fingers spread wide. Press the hips up into Downward-Facing Dog. Bend one knee toward the chest and press the ball of the foot down. Then begin to raise and lower the back leg, which stays straight, toes pointed. Pull the chest between the arms just as you do in Cobra pose. To gain the courage to kick up into a balance, work facing a wall and gaze ahead, not back, as you trust the momentum of your legs to swing your hips over your shoulders.

Man calls the peacock proud and vain. But the fantastic bird spreads its feathers to expand life force energy, oblivious to the beautiful spectacle it creates.

> Our only true course is to let the motive for action be in the action itself, never in its reward; not to be incited by the hope of the result, nor yet indulge a propensity for inertness.

—H. P. Blavatsky

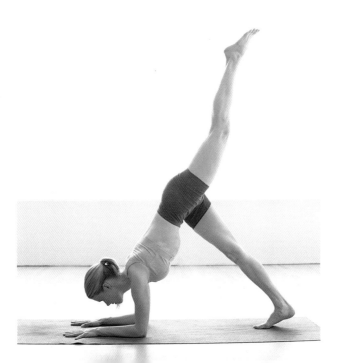

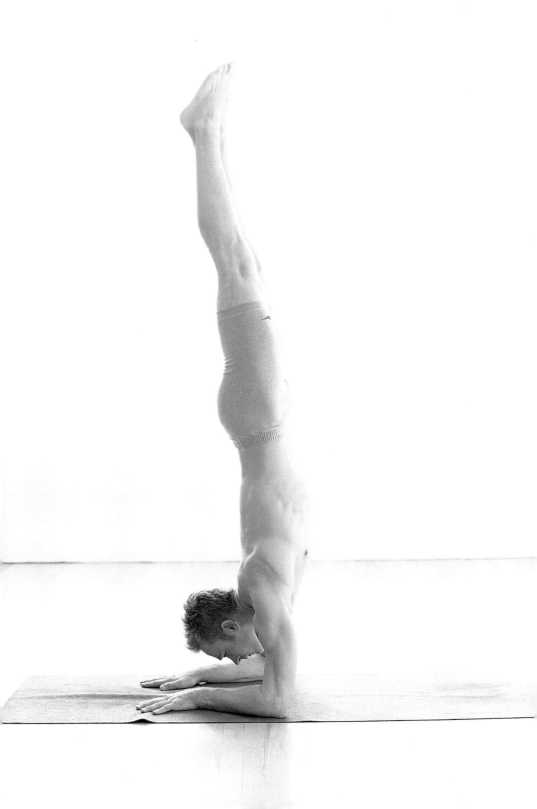

"Judge not, that ye be not judged," Jesus told his disciples. "For with what judgment ye judge, ye shall be judged; and with what measure ye mete it shall be measured to you again." The precepts of yoga also preclude judgment but stand this biblical teaching on its head a bit. Instead of "do unto others as you would have them do unto you," it's more "do unto others as you do unto yourself," a kind, practical approach.

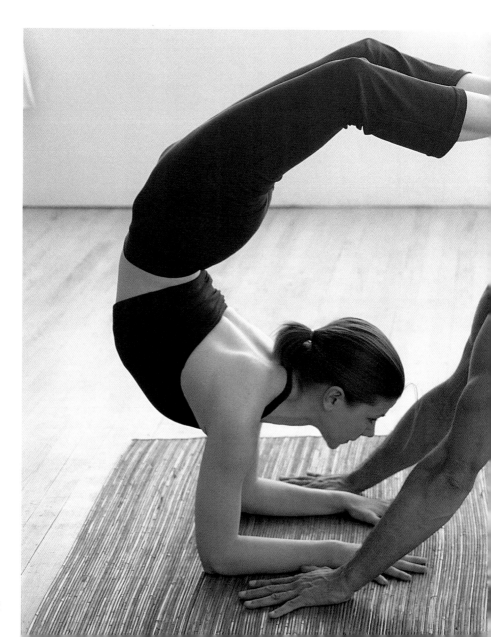

*If we can be pleased with those happier than ourselves, compassionate toward those who are unhappy, joyful with those doing praiseworthy things, and remain undisturbed by the errors of others, our minds will be tranquil.*

*—Yoga Sutras*

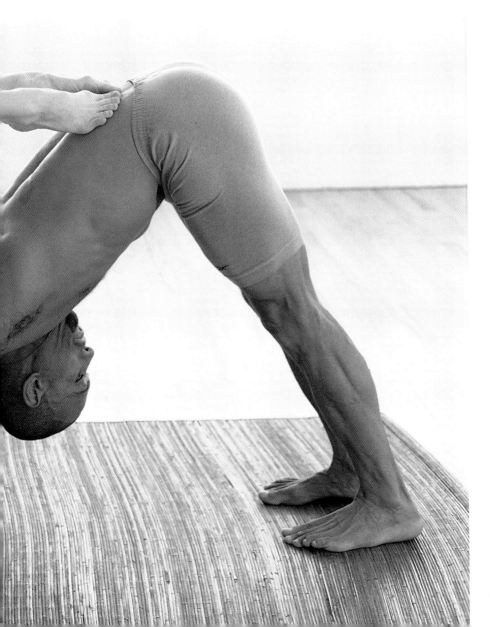

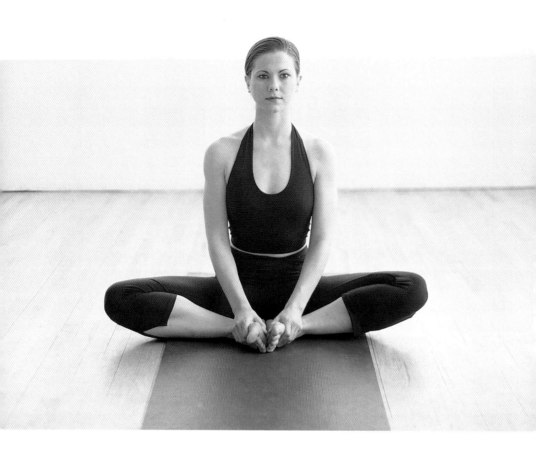

## Bound Ankle (Baddha Konasana)

Take the soles of your feet together and let the knees spread apart as they will. Press your palms into the floor behind you, wrists against sacrum and fingers facing away, and raise your buttocks off the floor until you feel length in the lower back. Then sit back down, maintaining that length as you move your hands to your feet. Holding the ankles, press your feet together with calm, intense energy, and feel how that translates into a lift in the sternum. Inhale deeply, and on an exhale pry the feet open like a book and bow forward, leading with the heart, not with the top of your head. Inhale again as you lengthen out, then exhale down and soften the neck wherever you are. Stay in the pose, breathing deeply into areas of resistance. Accept them; let them change.

A roomful of practitioners sitting in *Baddha Konasana*, or Cobbler's Pose, illustrates how differently we are all put together. Some people's knees fall splat out to the floor, while others' are practically up around their ears. Do not force your knees down; time and practice will ease them open.

**AHIMSA (NONHARMING):** How do you come to meet resistance? Providing plenty of it, hip openers like this are a laboratory for self-exploration. Notice how you play the edge of intense sensation. Do you hurtle toward it, then back away fast? Or do you tiptoe in overcautious, never risking the discomfort that accompanies change? Yogis develop the discretion to embrace the better part of both approaches by practicing *ahimsa*, nonviolence, which begins at home. Like your own good parent, patiently ride out fear and resistance, thereby cultivating the compassion that accommodates freedom—for yourself and for all beings.

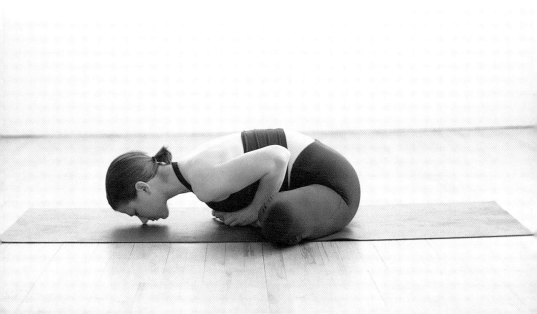

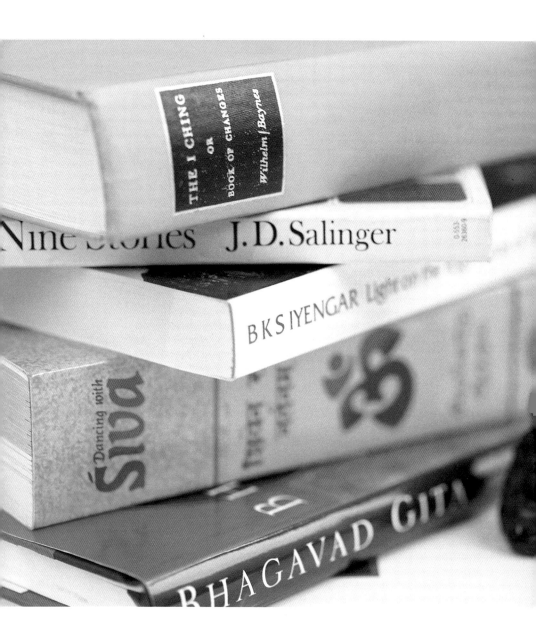

**SVADHYAYA (SELF-STUDY):**

*Read man; he is the living poem. We are the light that illumines all the Bibles and Christs and Buddhas that ever there were.*

*Go into your own room and get the Upanishads out of your own Self. Until the inner teacher opens, all outside teaching is in vain.*

—Swami Vivekananda

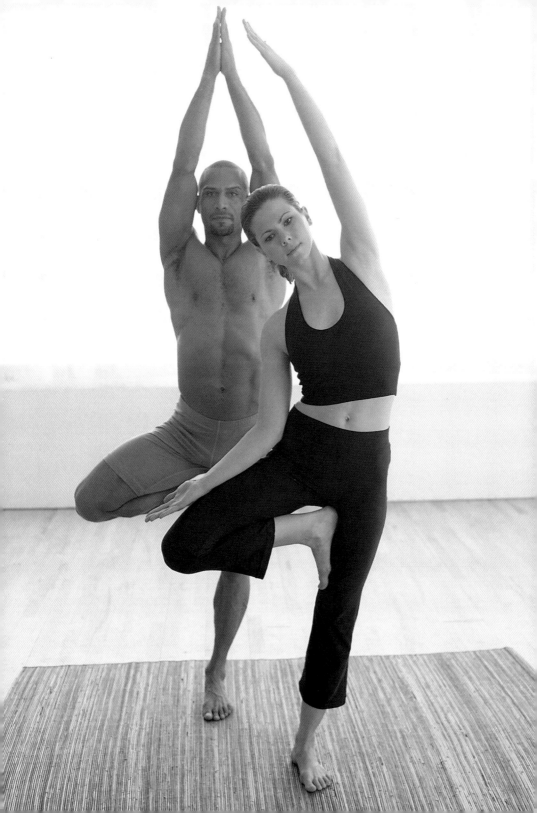

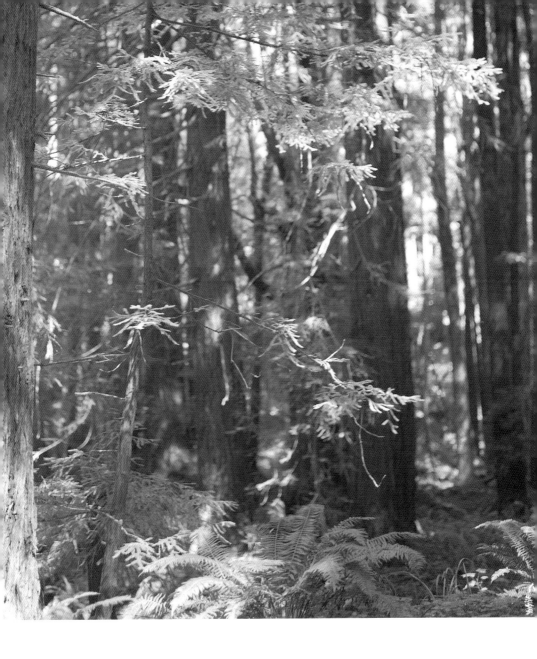

Trees are buffeted by winds all the time, and so are we. Unyielding limbs get snapped in two in a storm, but branches supple enough to bend withstand the harshest tempests. Tree pose (*Vrksasana*) teaches us not to cling to balance; it is not ours to begin with. Instead, we learn to ride the waves of motion and stillness.

Balance attained through self-sufficiency supports us alone and together.

# Locust (Salabhasana)

Lifting the back from a belly-down position is among the most strengthening exercises possible for the muscles along the spine. In addition, pressure to the abdominal region increases blood flow to the organs and improves digestion.

Lie on your abdomen with arms alongside the body, palms face up. Lift everything off the floor but the tops of your hands, sending the legs as much back as up and holding them straight and together. Don't crane the neck. To ensure that you lead with the chest and not with the head, gaze down the sides of your nose and move the shoulders down the back. Hold longer than you want to, breathing strongly and sweetly, then release.

# Bow (Dhanurasana)

Clasp your ankles and lift the chest and thighs off the floor, drawing the toes up and back. Prime your Bow for liberation; breathe confidently into the shape.

# Big-Toe Bow (Padangustha Dhanurasana)

A fuller expression of Bow pose.

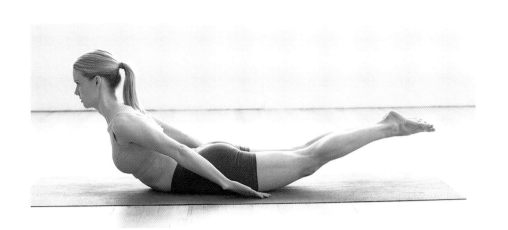

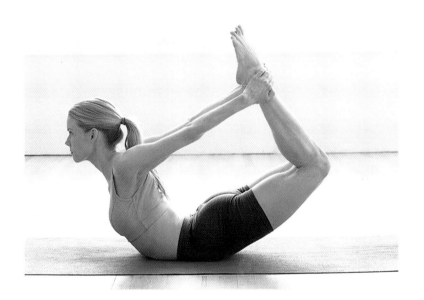

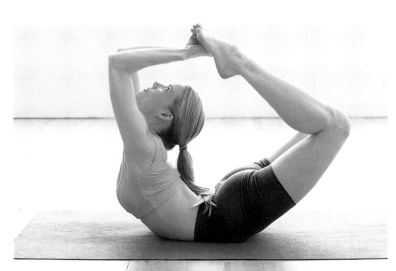

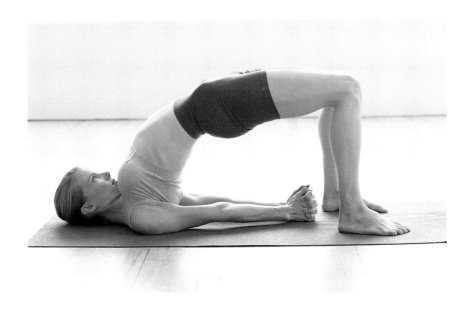

# Bridge or Half Wheel (Setu Bandhasana)

Lie on your back with knees bent and soles of the feet on the floor, heels hip-width apart and close to the sitting bones. Push into the feet to peel the spine up vertebra by vertebra, beginning with the tailbone, until your torso arcs toward the ceiling. Clasp your hands together beneath your back and wriggle the shoulders under the body.

Press the heels of the hands together to roll the upper arms out and to achieve lift between the shoulder blades, freeing the muscles around the thoracic spine. Send the knees forward over the toes, keeping the thighs active as if you are squeezing a beach ball between them. Inhale so deeply into the chest that it moves toward or to the chin. Lengthen from pubic bone to sternum.

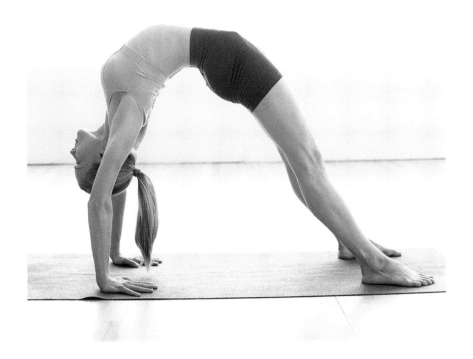

# Upward-Facing Bow or Full Wheel
## (Urdhva Dhanurasana)

Using the same alignment as for Half Wheel, place palms alongside ears, fingers under the shoulders and elbows over the wrists. When you are ready, press into the hands and feet and inhale smoothly up into Full Wheel. Keep your breathing calm and deep. Make certain the feet are parallel by turning the toes in a bit. When the feet splay out, the lower back constricts, shutting down the posture before it opens you up. Relax rather than thrust the pelvis; allow the sacrum to function as a broad tray that serves up the backbend. Let the lift derive from the legs, arms, and front of the body—and, as always, from the flow of *prana*, life force energy, within.

*Drink the cool beverage of contentment. Do not faint and fall in the rush owing to the feverish excitement of life and the intoxications of passion and power.*

—Swami Sivananda

**SANTOSA (CONTENTMENT):** Draw knees into chest to release the lower back and experience *santosa*, contentment, here, where it's easy, until you can elicit it in the deepest backbend.

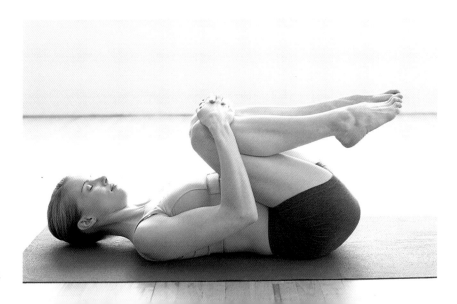

**BRAHMACHARYA** (**MODERATION**): One tenet of yoga philosophy not often literally observed, *brahmacharya* or adherence to chastity, nevertheless has broad implications for right living. To keep sacred what is sacred is a universal principle. By moderating our activity with care—in terms of *asana*, by tempering pose with counterpose—we become discriminating in what we send out and take in.

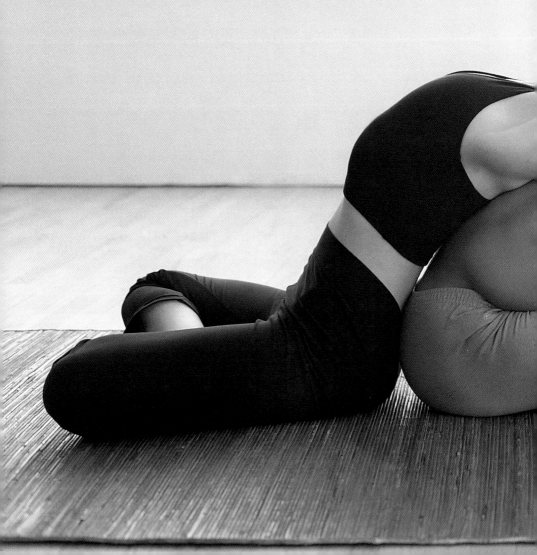

We cannot live if you and I have built a wall around ourselves and just peep over that wall occasionally. Unconsciously, deeply, under the wall, we are related.

—J. Krishnamurti

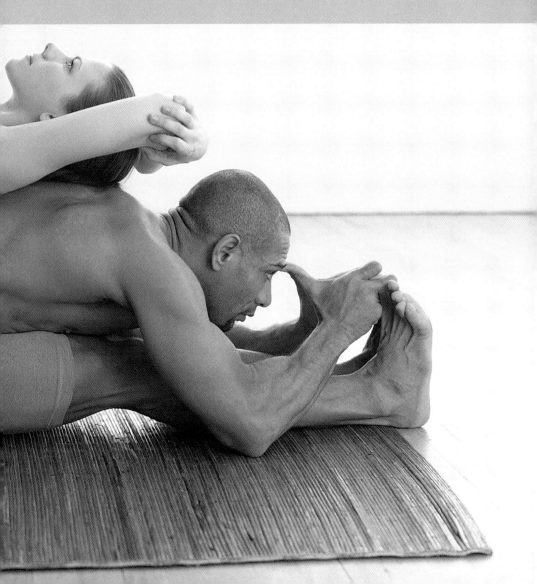

# Head-to-Knee (Janu Sirsasana)

Sit with the legs extended in front of you, feet flexed and torso lifted until the legs are strongly horizontal and the torso perfectly vertical. Open the right knee out ninety degrees, heel inside the right upper thigh. Square torso over the left leg.

On an inhale reach for the left foot or ankle and lift the chest, sending the shoulders down the back. Retain that openness in the front and back body as, on an exhale, you bow your heart—and then your head—to the knee.

The action of bowing, bringing the head lower than the heart, has always held great meaning for mankind. Used here as part of a posture, the gesture is also made in *yoga mudra* (bowing forward from any seated position) at an *asana* practice's conclusion, to seal in and proffer its benefits.

# Rotated Head-to-Knee (Parivrtta Janu Sirsasana)

Nestle the right shoulder inside the right thigh and reach the left arm up and overhead until you feel one long, expansive arch from the left sitting bone to the left middle finger. (Torso spins up, not down.) In this counterpose to *Janu Sirsasana*, we release the constriction of the abdominal organs, flooding the region with fresh oxygenated blood and energy.

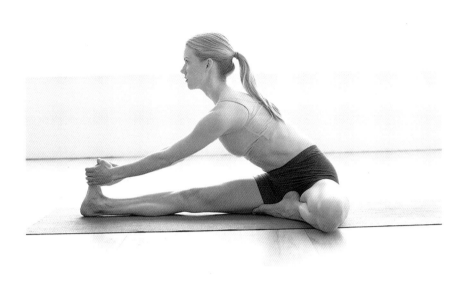

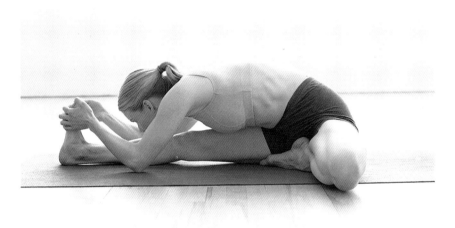

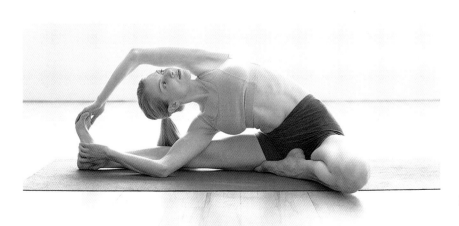

**ISVARAPRANIDHANA (DEVOTION):** Dedication of effort to *Isvara*, the eternal source, works to eradicate egoism, one of the causes of unhappiness cited by the Buddha and *Yoga Sutras* alike. Overassociation with one's separateness and the isolation that engenders are stumbling blocks on the path to yoga. So is the failure to acknowledge origin. In *asana* practice, do less. Let vitality course through you until you know in your bones that you are its instrument, not its instigator. Delve into the transcendental Self by consecrating the fruits of your labor.

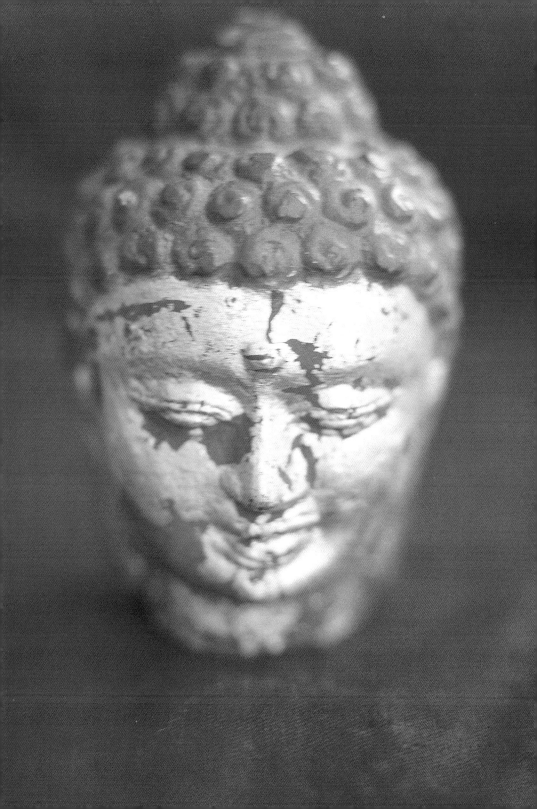

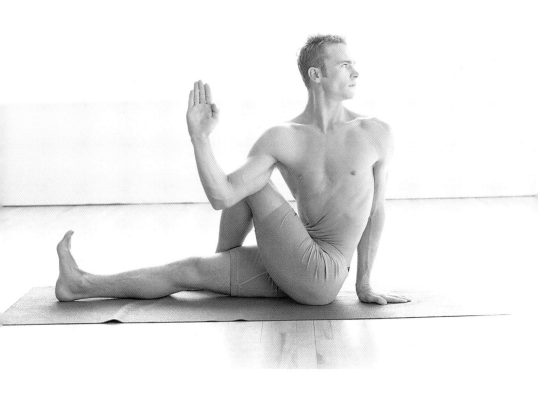

# Half-Seated Spinal Twist
(Ardha Matsyendrasana)

Sit with legs firmly extended in front of you. Bend left knee and place foot outside right knee. Position left arm behind you like a second spine— sit tall!—and hug or hook left knee with right elbow, spinning ribs, shoulders, and eyes to the left. Grow taller on each inhalation; twist more deeply on each exhalation. To bring the twist more toward the upper spine and shoulders, tuck the front leg back—but only if both sitting bones reach the floor—and thread top arm under the thigh to clasp the bottom wrist behind the back. To intensify work in the midback region, reach top hand over the knee and around the shin to clasp the ankle.

**AVIDYA (MISPERCEPTION):** In addition to massaging the internal organs and maintaining space and mobility in the spine and intervertebral discs, twists keep us supple in subtler ways. Remembering how—and why—to look around you wards off tunnel vision, the inability to change perspective. How many times have you seen a situation one way and been convinced you were right, only to find you were dead wrong? Through mindful *asana* practice, we remain pliant enough to minimize *avidya*, the incorrect perceptions that lead to personal and universal unhappiness.

How far you progress into a twist—or any posture—should be determined by your level of ease where you are. Follow the breath. Calm, strong inhalation and exhalation are safe passage to advancement.

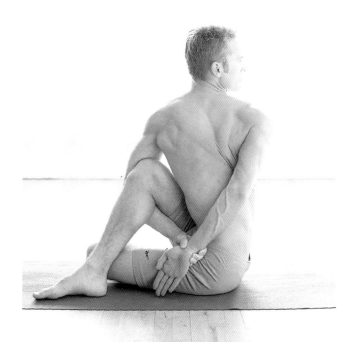

**SAUCHA** (**PURITY**): Cleanliness and purification inside and out— *tapas* and *saucha*, respectively—take natural priority as the body increasingly becomes the temple of the soul.

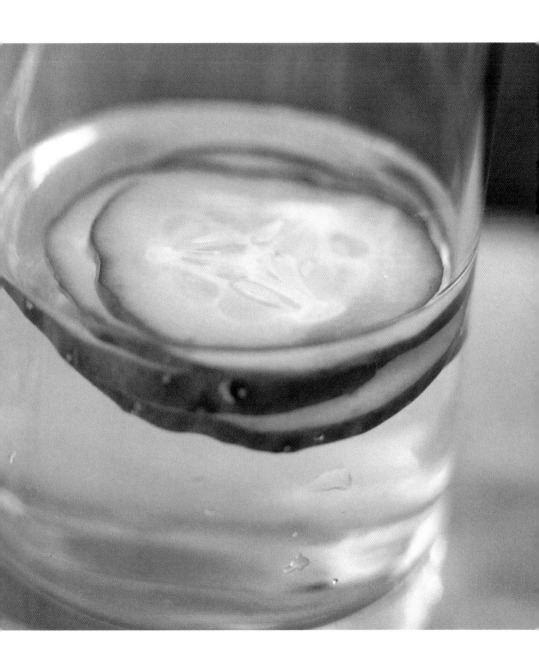

# Intense West or Back Stretch
## (Paschimottanasana)

Draw the flesh out from beneath the sitting bones and sit tall, legs together and actively extended. On an inhale lift the heart and reach toward whatever makes sense for you—the shins, the ankles, the big toes, or beyond. But do not become so fixed on what you are reaching for that you must hunch your back to attain it. Retain length in the lower back as you exhale into the forward bend, sending forehead or chin to the shins. Pull the navel toward spine on each exhalation and move more deeply into the pose.

Balance striving with receptivity here, being certain not to waste effort comparing yourself with anyone else. If tight hamstrings restrict you, try bending the knees to keep openness in the front and back body. If forward bending is easy, noncompetition becomes equally if not more important. Ward off hamstring injury by pulling the quadriceps up the thighs without locking the knees so the backs of the legs just come along for the ride. Pull the outer edges of the feet toward you with your fingers and press the tops of the big toe ball joints away with the thumbs. Once you have moved fully into the posture, relax the head and neck.

# Intense East or Front Stretch
## (Purvottanasana)

Place your palms on the floor eight to ten inches behind you, fingers facing buttocks. On an inhale, elevate the front of the body into a sort of reverse Upward-Facing Dog, with only the palms and soles of the feet touching the floor. Stretch all ten toes down and allow your head to fall back. If *Purvottanasana* is too difficult at first, do Tabletop: bend your knees and plant the feet beneath them, thrusting the pelvis up and keeping chin toward chest as your raise your hips high.

**S M R T I  (M E M O R Y ):** Intense forward bends engender reflection by bringing us up against limitations founded in the past. Be in the *Paschimottanasana* you are doing now, not the one you did yesterday or think you should be doing today. Soften into the fold; breathe memory into the present.

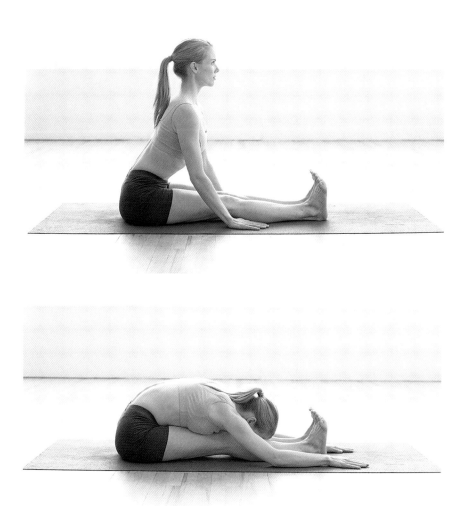

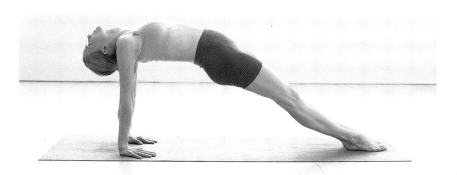

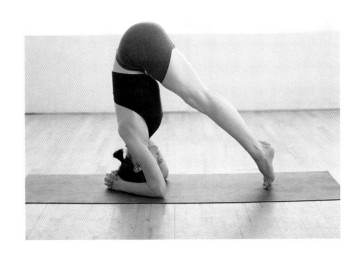

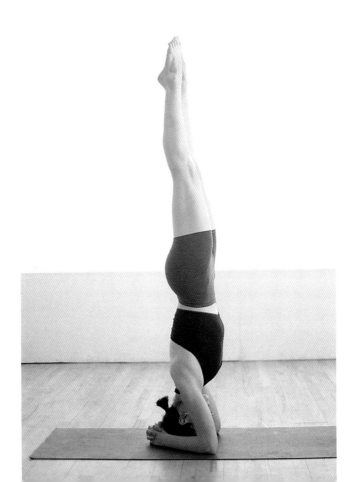

# Headstand (Salamba Sirsasana)

From a kneeling position, hug your elbows on the floor in front of you directly below your shoulders. Maintain that width as you extend the forearms straight out and interlace the fingers, making a loose basket. Place the top of your head on the floor and the back of your head in the basket. Tuck your toes under and press into a Downward-Facing Dog with your head on the floor, tiptoeing in until hips are directly over shoulders. This is Headstand practice. Work here until you understand what is required to bend one knee into the chest and then the other, taking the shape of an egg. Next, extend the legs to the ceiling, eventually learning to lift both legs straight up together. Press firmly into the pedestal you have created, dividing the weight among the elbows, forearms, and head. Move the shoulders away from the ears and squeeze your legs together, tightening the pelvic floor. Cull support from the intangible.

# Child Pose

Follow headstand practice with Child Pose. Sit on your heels and spill the torso over the thighs, forehead down and arms alongside the body so the shoulders melt to the floor.

Take a deep, full breath into the muscles of the back—and every now and then, hum your exhalation. The vibration of sound through the body, whether done simply or in chant (as on page 80), is powerful medicine.

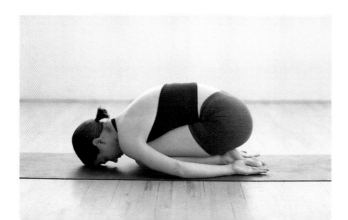

# DHARANA (CONCENTRATION):

*Arouse yourself to contemplate, to focus thought, for God is the annihilation of all thoughts, uncontainable by any concept.*

*—Kaballah*

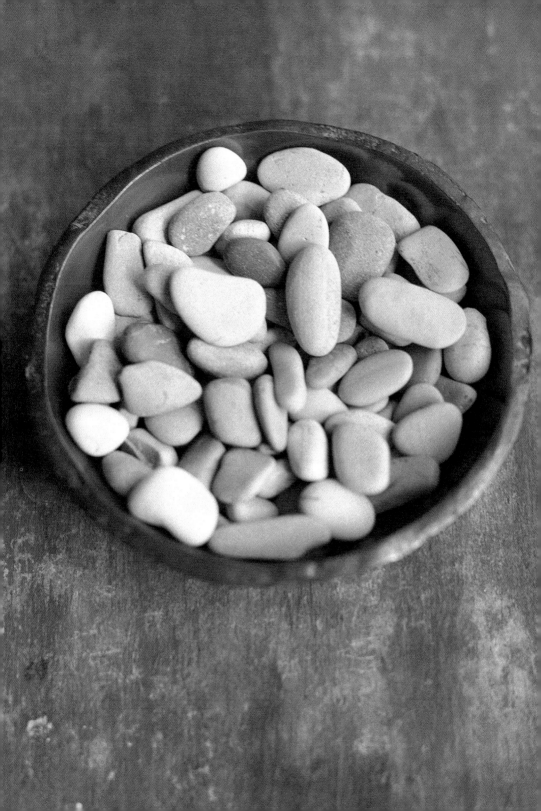

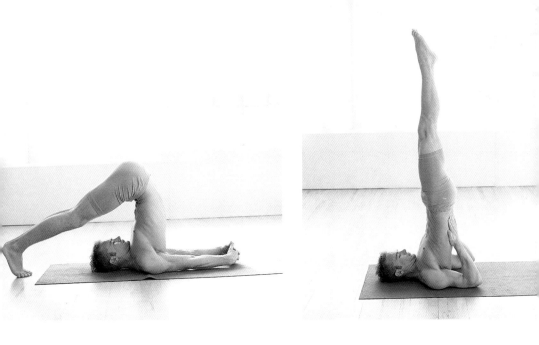

## Plow (Halasana)

Lying prone, bring the legs up and overhead so that the toes touch the floor behind you. (If they do not, try propping them up on a chair or block.) Press the heels away and the backs of the knees to the ceiling, aligning hips over shoulders. Interlace your fingers together behind the back, rolling the shoulders under and upper arms out. Find ease here before moving on.

## Shoulder Stand (Salamba Sarvangasana)

From *Halasana*, separate the hands and bend the elbows, bringing the palms to the back, fingers and thumbs together and facing up. Straighten one leg to the ceiling, then the other, keeping the inner legs active and the pelvis moving toward the face. Shoulder Stand gives the body a break from the pull of gravity, like all inversions. This traditional finishing posture for *asana* practice also stimulates glands in the head and neck, heightening endocrine system function. So build staying power into the pose. Distribute your weight among your shoulders, the back of your head (as opposed to the neck), and the arms and palms, which bolster the posture. If your neck is pressing into the floor, lie on a folded blanket with the shoulders at its edge and the head and neck extended beyond it. Choose and maintain one *drishti*—tip of the nose, navel, big toes, or between the brows with the eyes closed. Stay a minimum of fifteen slow breaths, then roll yourself down vertebra by vertebra, coming to lie flat with legs extended.

# Fish (Matsyasana)

Prop yourself on your elbows to sit up partway. On an inhale arch the entire spine—not just the upper back but the lower back, too—and as you exhale walk your fingers toward your heels until the top of the head is on the floor.

In this supported backbend, the counterpose to Shoulder Stand, we can inhale more completely than at any other time, breathing into the rarely oxygenated bases of the lungs. If it furthers the expansion to do so, press your palms in prayer and lift straightened arms and legs—feet pointed—off the floor at a forty-five degree angle.

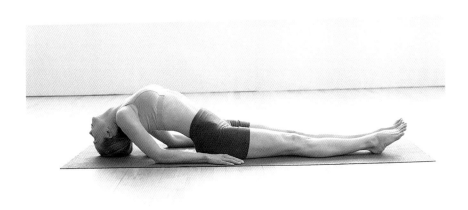

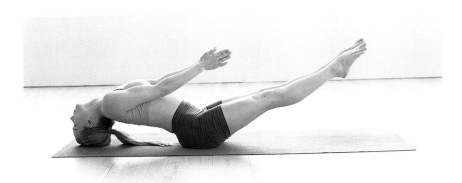

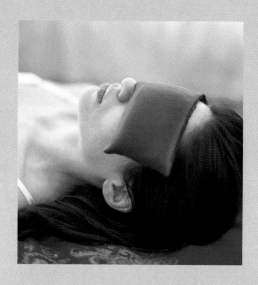

## PRATYAHARA (SENSE WITHDRAWAL):

*Take away the mental power from the external organs. You continually do it unconsciously when your mind is absorbed; so you can learn to do it consciously.*

—Swami Vivekenanda

# Corpse (Savasana)

*Asana* practice should always conclude with the conscious relaxation that is as much a posture as any active *asana*—and perhaps the most difficult to master. *Sava* means "corpse" in Sanskrit, and if that sounds macabre, it's not: the ancient yogis were interested in finding out what it's like when there is nothing left to do. So for as many minutes as possible, do nothing at all, and let everything happen.

Lie on your back with arms arranged comfortably alongside the body and feet splayed out, femur bones resting naturally in the hip sockets. Turn your palms to face the ceiling so the shoulders and heart can open. Close your eyes so the mind can open. Widen the sides of the throat so the soul can be free. Allow the forehead to smooth itself out. Then absolutely let go: Relax the bones and ligaments, the muscles that make your face your face, the thoughts that make you you. Come home to the strong, calm energy from which you were born, to which you will return, and of which you are made.

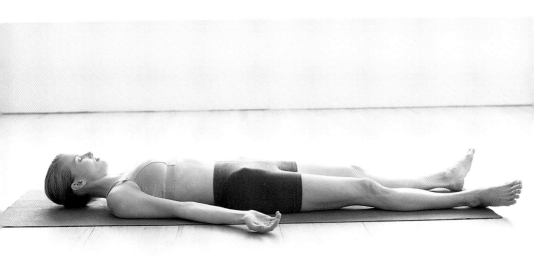

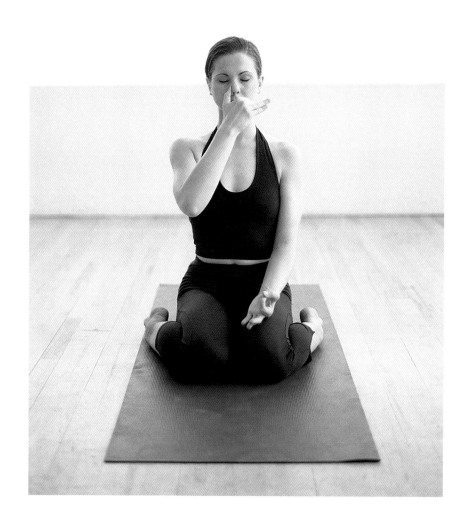

**PRANAYAMA (BREATH EXPANSION):** Integral to yoga practice is expanding the function of breath, once again by means of control. Here, too, that control must be nonviolent, "accompanied from the very beginning by feelings of peace and by soothing sensations of regenerative effect in the spine," instructed Paramahansa Yogananda, progenitor of yoga in the West. Breath retention practiced with *ahimsa* creates space, not restriction.

# Alternate Nostril Breathing (Nadi Sodhana)

The ancient yogis understood that bringing the left and right hemispheres of the brain into sync has a powerful effect on body and mind—the link between which is the breath. Curl the first two fingers of your right hand toward the palm and release the thumb, ring finger, and pinky. Inhale through both nostrils, then block off right nostril with thumb and exhale through the left side. Inhale through the left nostril, then block it off with the ring finger and pinky and exhale through the right. Inhale through the right, block off right nostril with thumb, and exhale through the left. Repeat three times with slow, deep, even breaths and no pause between the inhalation and exhalation. Then add retention to the mix: inhale through the left for a slow count of four seconds, block off both nostrils and retain for sixteen, exhale through the right for eight. Complete the cycle on the right side, then repeat entire sequence three times.

> *Conquest of the mind is more difficult than the conquest of the world by the force of arms. Become a hero. Conquer a formidable foe, this turbulent mind. Be regular in your meditation and come out victorious.*
>
> —Swami Sivananda

## Hero (Virasana)

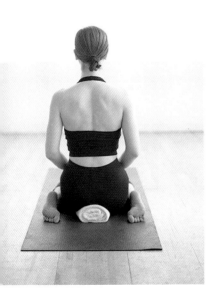

*Virasana* is a recommended seat for breathing exercises and meditation—which traditionally follow *asana* practice—so make yourself comfortable in this posture. Sit between your heels with knees together and tops of the feet on the floor alongside your hips. If you need padding to sit tall and still, roll up a towel, blanket, or yoga mat and insert the cylindrical shape from behind, between the sitting bones but not the thighs. If the tops of your feet hurt, pad there as well. After Hero pose, press gingerly or directly back to Downward-Facing Dog. These two postures in succession are tremendously therapeutic for the knee joints. Runners in particular should get to know and love this sequence.

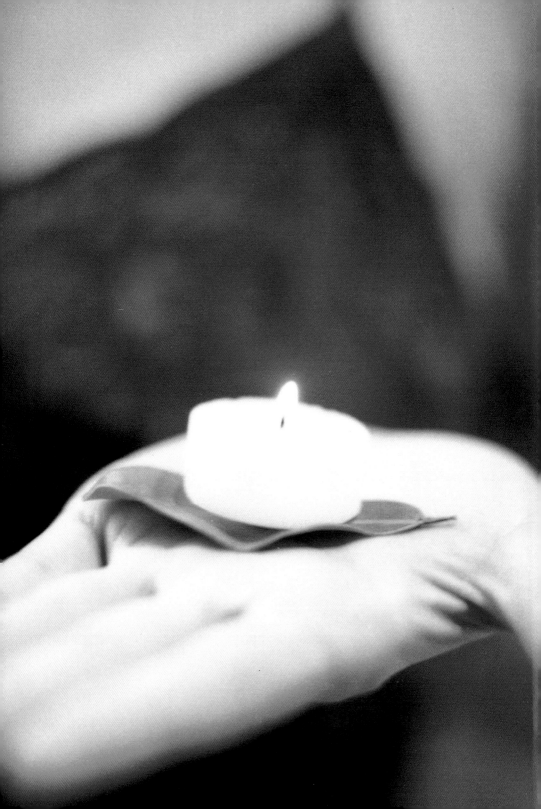

*The seeker of liberation should diligently effect the purification of the mind. When it is purified, liberation is as a fruit in one's hand.*

—*Amrita Bindhu Upanishad*


**DHYANA (MEDITATION):** Whether you have an active meditation practice, are just beginning one, or have little desire to try, you already know how to meditate. Animals and babies are past masters of the discipline, while most adult human beings engage in meditation only when they resolutely do not intend to—those random, surprising moments when your absorption in something is so complete you forget who you are. So do it intentionally, and teach yourself what you've always known.

The Buddha's instructions for meditation were simple: Breathing in, I know that I am breathing in; breathing out, I know that I am breathing out. Breathing in, I breathe my whole self in and so I train myself; breathing out, I breathe my whole self out and so I train myself.

The Vietnamese meditation master Thich Nhat Hahn, who urged his countrymen to practice *dhyana* while bombs and napalm dropped around them, offers a sweet addition: "Breathing in, I see myself as a flower; breathing out, I feel fresh. Breathing in, I see myself as a flower; breathing out, our hands, lips, eyes are flowers we give each other every day."

Take a comfortable seated position and direct your attention to the movement of the breath. When your mind wanders to matters great and small, return to observing the mechanism of respiration. The American Buddhist nun Pema Chödrön urges us to shepherd wandering attention back kindly, as you would a dear but fractious child. "Without making any big deal whatsoever, simply come back... developing a nonaggressive attitude to whatever goes on in your mind," she advises. In meting out such loving-kindness to ourselves, Chödrön counsels, we cannot help but spread it around.

At the conclusion of *asana* practice, meditation becomes most effortless. You have used virtually all your muscles, worked the joints, and twisted your body this way and that, opening the channels of energy and stilling the mind. "*Tada drashtu svarupe 'vasthanam,*" the *Sutras* explain and we come to discover: Now the Seer, the true Self, is seen. And the glimpses of bliss, or *samadhi*, that have taunted us all our lives become a *drishti* we choose to maintain.

Salute the light within you and without you.
*Namaste.*

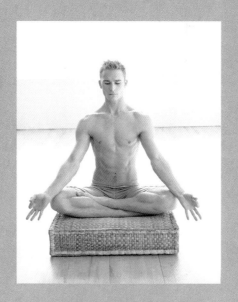

*asato maa sadgamaya*
*tamaso maa jyotir gamaya*
*mrityor maa amrtam gamaya*
*om shanti, shanti, shanti.*

Lead me from the unreal to the real,
from ignorance to knowledge,
from death to immortality.
Om. Peace, peace, peace.